50+ Business Ideas for the Entrepreneurial Nurse

Nachole Johnson

Copyright 2016 Nachole Johnson and ReNursing Publishing Company.

ALL RIGHTS RESERVED.

ISBN: *1539426912*

ISBN-13: 978-1539426912

Disclaimer

Although the author and publisher have made every effort to ensure the information provided in this book were correct at press time, the author and publisher do not assume and hereby disclaim any liability to any party for any loss, damage, or disruption caused by errors or omissions, whether such errors or omissions result from negligence, accident, or any other cause.

This book is not intended as the substitute for the legal advice or consultation of attorneys. The reader should regularly consult an attorney in matters relating to his/her business that may require legal advisement.

All rights are reserved. No part of this publication may be reproduced, distributed, more transmitted in any form or by any means, including photocopying, recording, or other electronic or means, including photocopying, recording, or any other electronic or mechanical methods, without the prior written permission of the publisher, except in no commercial use permitted uses permitted by copyright law.

TABLE OF CONTENTS

Introduction

My Story

Chapter 1 Why You Should Read This Book

Chapter 2 Creative Arts Businesses
Medical Photographer
Medical Writer
Resume Writer/Reviewer
Nurse Artist
Mobile Painting Party Service
Medical Interior Designer
Medical Product Reviewer
Medical Researcher / Writer

Chapter 3 Educational Businesses
NCLEX Review Instructor
Nursing School Tutor
BLS and ACLS Instructor
Educational Vacation Seminars
Medical Spanish for Healthcare Providers Instructor
CE Online Bank or Registry
ESL instructor
Nurse Consultant

Chapter 4 Child Services Businesses
After-hours Daycare
Mobile School Nurse
In-hospital Daycare Center
Sick Daycare Center
Nanny Referral Agency
Adoption Escort Services
Home Safety Assessment Nurse

Chapter 5 Skills Businesses
Foot Care Nurse
PICC/Midline Insertion Nurse
EKG Instructor
CNA School
Skills Training Workshop
Phlebotomy School

Chapter 6 Travel Businesses
Vacation Companion Travel Nurse Agency
Medical Transport
Mobile Flu Vaccine Clinic
Mobile Infusion (Hang-Over Clinic)
Public Speaker

Chapter 7 Tech Savvy Businesses
Website or Domain Flipper
Medical Website Designer
App Developer
Podcaster

Chapter 8 Health and Wellness Businesses
Health and Wellness Spa
Fitness studio
Pre/intra/post-natal fitness instructor
Massage Nurse

Chapter 9 Care-giving Businesses
Patient Advocate
Case Manager
Group Home Owner
Pet Therapy Service
Home Health Agency
Assisted Living Facility
Elder Daycare

Chapter 10 Miscellaneous Businesses
Medical Supply Retail Store
Stock Investor
Real Estate Investor
Inventor
Franchise
Crime Scene Clean Up Service
Nursing Staffing Agency
Expert Witness Nurse
Subscription Box Service

Chapter 11 What Next?
How to ensure your business is profitable
Dealing with discouragement
How to Raise Capital for Your Business

About the Author

Other Books By Nachole Johnson

You're a Nurse and Want to Start Your Own Business? The Complete Guide. Available at https://www.amazon.com/dp/B00H4OVHKC/

Introduction

Over the years, I have encountered many nurses who have become dissatisfied with their jobs for various reasons. The long hours, physical labor, and constant multitasking on a daily basis gets tiring. They always have the option of working in a clinic, but that also poses challenges for some nurses. The biggest complaints I hear about clinic work is the low pay and having to work five days a week instead of three.

Before I started my own business, I had imagined for years what type of business I could start with my nursing experience. I racked my brain for the longest before I decided what I could do on a daily basis that I would enjoy (and make money from!) This is where my inspiration for my first book came from. *You're a Nurse and Want to Start Your Own*

Business? The Complete Guide covers a broad range of business topics related to nurses like how to pick the right business. It also outlines the steps needed to start and maintain a successful business.

For many of the nurses I counsel about starting their own business, I find that brainstorming a business idea is one of their greatest struggles. The second most common issue is start-up costs. They typically do not want or cannot afford high start-up costs. Since you are reading this book, I assume you have the same problem. I am here to help you. The businesses in this book have a range of start-up costs from the bare minimum to tens of thousands. The costs just depend on where your passion lies with the sort of business you want to pursue.

This book is a compilation of different business ideas for the entrepreneurial nurse. I have broken down the career ideas by specific categories such as: creative careers, travel careers, consulting careers, etc. Each career also has information on additional education required, how much to expect for start-up costs, whether or not you can pursue this business by brick & mortar, online, or travel, and potential products and services you can upsell in the business.

This book will not include state and location specific guidelines to pursue your business of choice. This is something you will have to research on your own. I do not and cannot attest to the specifics to carry out every business venture. Some businesses listed will take the partnership of a medical doctor depending on your educational background (LPN, RN, APRN) and the state where you intend to do business.

If possible, I suggest finding a mentor who can help you start your specific business venture. In addition, you will also not find specific, but only potential start-up costs for each business. I am providing you with potential costs that include setting up your business from a legal perspective. I cannot foresee the amount of supplies, licensing, permits, and other fees are for your particular area. Take this book as guidance on how you can capitalize from your nursing education, but do not assume it is a covers everything you may need.

My hope for this book is that after you finish reading it you will have a solid idea of a business you can pursue for yourself. If for any reason you need more assistance with starting your own business or brainstorming a particular idea, feel free to contact me through my career consulting website www.renursing.com or email me at info@renursing.com

My Story

During my 15 years as a nurse, the profession has failed me in several ways. As a nurse, I thought I would never be out of a job and would be able to get a job anywhere. For the most part, what I envisioned was true. In my earlier years, I had a steady job and did not have much difficulty finding another job if need be within my specialty.

Over time I became disillusioned with the profession because I was not making the money up I thought I deserved as an experienced nurse. I stayed with a company and did not receive a raise for most of the seven years I was there. I started to hate my job, not only because my pay was not fair, but because of the exhaustion, the crap tasks nurses were expected to complete, the endless disrespect from doctors, patients, and management. The list of why I began to dislike nursing was starting to pile up, and I was miserable.

At that time, I tried to find an exit plan to get out, or at least make my life better. I figured I'd go for the money. I thought, "I can tolerate anything for the right price." Boy, was I wrong! I pursued anesthesia school for the money, but I crashed and burned from the sheer stress, and accumulated an enormous student loan debt.

After that experience, I went to Nurse Practitioner school and chose the FNP route because I thought it would be the most marketable. Well, that did not apply to the Houston market! Starting salaries were crazy low – I mean like 85k. I could have made that without overtime as an RN – on day shift. "Pffft..." I thought, "You want me to be a provider, diagnosing and treating, with all the liability of physicians but still make less than a third of what they do? Yea, right. No way, Jose."

That is why I shifted into the health and wellness realm of my nurse practitioner career. My first job was teaching patients about Metabolic Syndrome and its effects on future health outcomes. I loved that job, but it was only on a per diem basis, not enough to sustain a sufficient income.

Soon afterward, I took a position as a Center Director of an infusion center. The job sounded great at first. I was a manager and had the responsibility of opening the first clinic of its kind in my area.

I soon burned out from that job. I was the sole employee and had to do everything. I had to check patients in and out, verify their insurance, do a complete history and physical on each patient, start their IV, and administer their medication. I also answered the phone; set up the clinic with furniture and organized everything, ordered and checked in medications and supplies. I also had to be on call seven days a week for new patients coming in. I was effectively running a business for someone else! How crazy was that?

I ended up with constant tension, begging management for help, but to no avail. Finally, the pressure damaged my health so that I needed major surgery. My boss quickly asked if I needed the full six weeks off after a major surgery. She did not want to hire anyone else to cover me for the six weeks I would be gone. Sadly, I was looking forward to having surgery so I could have six weeks of rest from that job! Soon after my return, I gave my notice because I just could not handle the stress. She finally granted permission to hire a couple of employees (after more begging and reminding my boss how unsafe it was to be the only person in the clinic). I put in my notice three months after I returned to work.

After that job, I worked as much as I could at my favorite NP job. A few months later, I landed a job, making Medicare home visits, doing assessments on the geriatric population. The job was great for the first month and a half, but then my patient load dropped. I was a full-time NP with the company, but I was not getting enough patients to sustain a steady income. One week, I only had seven patients on my schedule when I was supposed to see 25! You can imagine how horrible my paycheck looked.

The shortage of patients continued, and my personal finances were strapped because of medical expenses from the previous year's surgery. Complaints to management landed on deaf ears. Maybe they knew what was going on and just didn't care. In desperation, I scrambled to find another job.

I found one shortly before the company laid me off due to lack of patients. This job only lasted five months. My next position was in wellness, and it was also amazing, or so I thought. I ended up being laid off because the company was too disorganized to know how to manage their money. I was laid-off only after three and one-half months on the job. The company closed three out of their nine locations, and I just so happened to be in one of the lucky clinics. They gave us no warning of the layoff; they just came in and let us go– with no severance pay. I wasn't there long enough to collect unemployment from the state. I was screwed once again as an NP. Luckily, I had about four months of savings at this point, so it wasn't too bad of a financial hit. I was just getting back on my feet from the previous underemployment and job loss a few months before.

At this point, I decided to go for my own business. I didn't have much in my overall retirement accounts because I had been underpaid. My last job didn't even offer retirement benefits. These small setbacks were messing up my financial future. I had been laid off two separate full-time positions in healthcare within four 1/2 months of each other. By this time, I didn't trust any employer to help me become financially secure. Let's face it, I had a job on Monday and was laid off on Tuesday without warning. Where is the security many so called loyal employees tout? I was over it at this point.

I had always wanted to start my own business and do something big, but like so many others, I was afraid. After losing two jobs in a row, my fear dissolved. I figured I was better off doing my own thing and hedging my bets in business. Now, I seriously began to explore options to become a serious business owner. I was finally serious about it.

I believe a series of events brought me to this path. Maybe a traditional work path was not for me. I share my story not to discourage anyone from nursing or to push my views on anyone else. I share because I know it is possible to follow your dreams and make something for yourself. My hope is that this book will help someone achieve his or her full potential.

Chapter 1
Why You Should Read This Book

Are you tired of not being able to eat, drink, or even pee while you are at work? What about working weekends and holidays? Have you ever missed a family function (child's recital, graduation, etc) because you had to work? Do you feel like you are paid much less than you are worth? I am sure you have answered yes to many, if not all, of these questions at some point in your nursing career. It gets exhausting after a while, doesn't it?

You are reading this book because you want a change.

There are many reasons nurses want to break free from traditional nursing and start their own business. You may have your own reasons for starting your own business, but you may be stuck on what you should do or where to start. Many nurses have this problem. They do not think their nursing skills are translatable to any other career, let alone starting their own business. I wrote this book to prove them wrong. Nursing skills are translatable to other careers, especially business!

I know nursing schools do not educate us on starting our own businesses. When I was brainstorming for my own business, I realized the sad reality that I don't know anything but nursing! However, being the ambitious, enterprising person that I am, I began to research business. I read books; I joined online groups; I started seeking out like-minded people; and—I started a business.

All my research and life experience about business came together in my first book: *You're a Nurse and Want to Start Your Own Business? The Complete Guide.* I thought I had a complete guide for my fellow nursing buddies, but I missed one important thing: many nurses would love to start their own business, but most have no clue of what type of business to start! I gave them all the information to get a business started, but I did not offer many ideas for my readers to bounce around. That is where this book comes in.

Some people do not realize you can turn your hobbies and passions into a viable and profitable business! How fun would it be to create a business from a hobby? This book is filled with much more than those run-of-the-mill hobby-type businesses. I've brainstormed over 50 businesses nurses can easily transition into with their education ranging from hobbies to make a little bit of cash on the side to full-fledged nursing enterprises. Are you ready to find the perfect business idea? All right! Let's go!

Chapter 2
Creative Arts Businesses

Medical Photographer

So you have a passion for photography? If you do, you can turn your hobby into a business and profit from it! I am not talking taking photos for weddings or birthday parties. You can still do that if you like, but I have developed a way for you to be much more profitable as a photographer while using your nursing background.

How does this relate to nursing you may ask? A nurse could easily establish a business as medical photographer. A medical photographer takes pictures of surgical procedures, medical devices and pictures for the company newsletter. This job would normally be as a freelancer. Big companies do not like keeping people on staff and paying them a full-time salary and benefits when they can save money by bringing someone in occasionally to do the job. That's where you come in. You will automatically be cheaper because you have no overhead. As a freelance medical photographer, you come in take photos, get paid, and repeat. It is as simple as that!

If you enjoy taking photos for fun and want to get into medical photography, start working on your portfolio. It would also be beneficial if you had some kind of experience in working with Photoshop and other photo editing software.

There are classes for photography, but I know of many self-taught photographers. The main selling point for whether or not someone will hire you is going to be your portfolio.

Additional Resources:
BioCommunications Association.
http://www.bca.org
Health Sciences Communications Association.
http://www.hesca.org

Potential Start-up costs: $500 or less (not including equipment)

Additional degree required: No

Sole venture or partnership: Sole

Mobile, Online, or Brick & Mortar: Mobile

Potential products to upsell: Photo editing, graphic layouts, photographing at social events

Medical Writer

Are you a nurse who likes writing? Did you know you could combine the two and start a profitable business? Writing is a creative industry. How much creativity do you get to have on your day job now? Not much as a nurse. However, being a nurse can help you be a better writer.

The experience you have as a nurse can translate into a specific kind of writing. You can market yourself as a medical writer. As a medical writer, you will write about various medical subjects for trade magazines, hospitals, books and even movie and TV scripts!

In this context, you would set yourself up as a freelance writer, just as the medical photographer does. Like a medical photographer, there is usually no additional degree required. Being the wonderful, hardworking nurse you are is enough!

As a freelance medical writer, you set your own hours to work. You can work from home or at the local coffee shop. There are deadlines for writing projects to be completed, but this is no different from any other job. You also set your own fees as a freelancer. Write, submit, are paid, and repeat.

You need very little to set up shop as a freelance writer. Items needed include a computer, paper, pencils, and your business license.

Additional Resources:
American Medical Writers Association
http://www.amwa.org

Freelance Writer's Den
http://www.freelancewritersden.com

Potential Start-up costs: $500 or less (not including equipment)

Additional degree required: No

Sole venture or partnership: Sole

Mobile, Online, or Brick & Mortar: Brick & Mortar

Potential products to upsell: Writing your own book, offering copyediting services, writing for blogs and magazines, or writing for different industries.

Resume Writer/Reviewer

As someone who has experience with hiring (and sometimes firing) people, I have to say that the way your resume is written says a lot about you. Many nurses don't understand how to present themselves in a resume. As a result, even excellent nurses are often overlooked for interviews because their resume is poorly written.

If you have a knack for grammar and know how to create a killer resume, then resume writing may be for you. Resume writing provides an important service to all involved. It captures and holds the attention of the interviewer. It is often what gets the nurse into the door for an interview. The more interviews a person gets, the greater possibility they will land a desirable job. See? It is a win-win situation for everyone.

Resume writing/reviewing does not involve much in the way of start-up costs and can be done in the comfort of your own home.

Additional Resources:
Professional Association of Resume Writers
http://www.parw.com

National Resume Writers Association-
http://www.thenrwa.com

Potential Start-up costs: $500 or less (not including certification-which is not required, but adds to your value).

Additional degree required: No

Sole venture or partnership: Sole

Mobile, Online, or Brick & Mortar: Online

Potential products to upsell: Cover letter services, interview coaching.

Nurse Artist

Just because you are a nurse doesn't mean you aren't a creative soul at heart. Many nurses have a talent for art and don't know that they can capitalize from it. I enjoy painting and didn't think of making a career of art!

If you enjoy painting, sculpting, woodworking, scrapbooking, etc—you name it—you can do it as a career. I've come across some very creative types in the medical field. Creativity is not something that can be learned, but your innate artistic talent can be honed and perfected. If your artistic work is good, someone will be willing to pay you for it!

If you are an artistic type, start building a portfolio of your best pieces and begin to show them at galleries, art festivals, and on your own website. The more exposure the better! As an artist, you can sell your work at any of these venues—at any price you want. Your earning potential is unlimited to what someone is willing to pay for your art.

If you are an artist of some type, you probably have all you need to get your business off the ground. All you really need to start out with is a good website to display your work.

Additional Resources:
Art by Nurses http://www.artbynurses.com
JParadisi RN's Blog http://jparadisirn.com

Potential Start-up costs: $100 or less (not including art supplies)

Additional degree required: No

Sole venture or partnership: Sole

Mobile, Online, or Brick & Mortar: Online

Potential products to upsell: Picture books featuring your art, various items with your art imprinted (t-shirts, mugs, etc), posters.

Mobile Painting Party Service

This career venture will appeal to the artistic nurse as well, though you aren't selling your own art – you're selling the artist experience to partygoers.

This business is similar to the Paint and Sip studios that have popped up all over the U.S. in the last few years. The premise is to throw a party that allows the partygoers to create their own masterpiece in the comfort of a private home instead of a studio. This type of business would cater to bachelorette parties, baby showers, and children's birthday parties.

Additional Resources: Get an example at: https://www.gigmasters.com/face-painting/artme

Potential Start-up costs: $500 or less (not including art supplies)

Additional degree required: No

Sole venture or partnership: Sole

Mobile, Online, or Brick & Mortar: Mobile

Potential products to upsell: Same products as "Nurse Artist" including your own original pieces of work.

Medical Interior Designer

Do you have a great sense of design and HGTV just happens to be your favorite channel? Why not use you design skills to help remodel hospital units and nurses' stations? Did you know that the interior design field needs nurses who can help with layouts of hospitals, nursing homes, and other medical facilities?

Architectural firms hire nurses for insight on these types of jobs on a consultant basis. You could even take it a step further and obtain your degree in Healthcare Design as an interior designer so you will be the one actually drawing up the sketches and plans for designs.

This is a harder field to break into as a nurse, but it can be done. You may have to use your networking skills to find others in the field and make a niche for yourself. Start attending networking meeting with architectural firms; call local hospitals to see if they have nurses on staff who do this. The name of the job varies depending on the facility, so it may take a bit of digging around to find what you are looking for.

Additional Resources: University of Minnesota Healthcare Design and Innovation post-Baccalaureate Certificate
https://www.nursing.umn.edu/degrees-programs/certificates/health-care-design-and-innovation-post-baccalaureate-certificate

Nursing Institute for Healthcare Design
http://www.nursingihd.com

Potential Start-up costs: $0- Unknown, depending if you go back to school for a design degree

Additional degree required: Yes, in most cases

Sole venture or partnership: Sole

Mobile, Online or Brick & Mortar: Brick & Mortar, but may require extensive travel

Potential products to upsell: Arbitrage of other services such as architectural and custom furniture designs. These can be outsourced to others for the actual work, with you doing the sourcing and supervision.

Medical Product Reviewer

This business involves having your own website for reviews, but also posting copies of your reviews on other sites as well. It combines several skills, including writing ability and photography. You will be writing review articles and including photos of medical equipment, clothing, and supplies (not pharmaceuticals). It is not necessary for you to purchase these items. You can begin by writing a collection of reviews of products and equipment you use daily at work. Be honest about the strengths and weaknesses of each item because this will build your credibility.

It will be a slow beginning, but it also has very low start-up costs. This venture is ideal for a part-time start while you keep your day job. After getting a website designed and learning how to post blog entries, you can begin evaluating products at work. Later, you can contact manufacturers to see if they are interested in having their products reviewed on your site and on related sites or social media groups. Give them your credentials and why you selected them for review. If they agree, normally they will send you samples to try out. In some cases, these items will be useful to you at work or could be sold online to add more income. Beware, however, some items cannot be posted on sites like Amazon without having a special license to do so. As one example, CPAP machines have these restrictions.

One of the most important keys to success will be building a large email list to help drive traffic to your site. You will need to develop free offers to get visitors to subscribe to your site. Post on social media groups related to the medical profession as well.

Additional Resources: Here are some sample websites:
Verywell.com
https://www.verywell.com/medical-product-reviews-4013439

Whichmedical device.com
http://www.whichmedicaldevice.com/

Potential Start-up costs: $0 if you can set up your own website. Up to $200 if you can't.

Additional degree required: No

Sole venture or partnership: Sole.

Mobile, Online or Brick & Mortar: Online

Potential products to upsell: Sidebar ads on your website can be offered to suppliers and manufacturers (after you have enough traffic). You may also contact local medical supply stores. Offer free ads to your first ten advertisers.

Medical Researcher / Writer

Maybe you are one of those people who actually love researching new things online or at the library. Maybe you like to write summaries of your findings or to develop a bibliography showing all your sources. Even if you might be ashamed to admit being a geek, you could become a prosperous one!

This idea can be developed in several ways. You could save doctors time by researching the latest information on a disease, medication, or procedure. You could do research for medical or other healthcare students who are writing a thesis or other paper. I assure you, the demand will be high! The most important part of the process is the same as other businesses, marketing your service. That can be done through social media to attract users to your website. Yes, you will need one of those! You can also begin the process through freelance websites.

Your overhead will be almost nonexistent until you start hiring others to join you. Then, you might need to supply desks and computers. You will need internet access. Eventually, you'll want to subscribe to sites that offer access to many resources at a single location. Databases like the EBSCO Medline Complete are very expensive, but as your business grows, it could be a great timesaver.

You can hire your researchers from the obvious sources – colleges and university students who don't want to be strangled with student loan debt. You will need to establish standards for them and a screening process for hiring, but this business could rapidly expand.

Additional Resources: For examples:

https://www.upwork.com/o/jobs/browse/?q=Medical Writing

Potential Start-up costs: $0 to $100.

Additional degree required: No

Sole venture or partnership: Either

Mobile, Online or Brick & Mortar: Online

Potential products to upsell: Annotated outlines of research papers. The student still writes the paper, but the material is completely organized for them. BIG MONEY!

Nachole Johnson

Chapter 3
Educational Businesses

NCLEX Review Instructor

Does graduation from nursing school make you a nurse? No! You have to take the NCLEX! All nursing students who graduate from school need to take the NCLEX, don't they? Yes! An experienced nurse who loves to teach can use this to their advantage.

I'm sure you have fond memories of graduating from school but weren't relieved because you still had to pass the NCLEX before you could start working as a nurse. You can help graduate nurses qualm their fears and ace that exam by becoming an NCLEX review instructor.

Obviously, you know how to pass the NCLEX because you are a nurse already! In order to start an NCLEX review business, you would need to stay abreast of the current NCLEX guidelines to ensure your students are well prepared for the exam. Study the current guidelines by reading NCLEX review books and visit the official NCLEX accrediting body.

NCLEX reviews can be carried out online or in person, so this business has the potential to be very lucrative. Online courses can be recorded so you don't have to present the course live. That is an automatic way to make money while you sleep! An NCLEX review instructor could also offer 1-on-1 tutoring services for an additional price. The possibilities are endless of how this business could grow and become profitable!

To start your own NCLEX review course you need to spend some time developing course materials for your students (course curriculum, manuals, etc.) You will also need to determine if you want to do strictly online courses or in person sessions. I use the online platform Udemy for courses. It is easy to set up your course and you receive 70% profit from each sale. As the course instructor, you determine your own pricing for each course. A sweet deal if I don't say so myself!

Additional Resources:
Dr. Johnson-Umez NCLEX Review Course for RNs and LVNs
http://www.nclexreviewcourse.com

Rinehart & Associates Nursing Review
http://www.nclexreview.net

Potential Start-up costs: $1,000 or less

Additional degree required: No

Sole venture or partnership: Either

Mobile, Online or Brick & Mortar: Any

Potential products to upsell: Your own NCLEX review material, offering 1-on-1 tutoring, online review courses, audio review materials, developing other nursing-related courses

Nursing School Tutor

Was nursing school hard for you? Do you remember struggling through, worrying if you would pass your next exam or not? I sometimes had these thoughts while in school. Having a personal tutor during school would have helped me tremendously. I'm sure I am not the only one who has had these thoughts, and I'll bet my last dollar that current nursing students are going through the same thing.

Why not help the new nursing generation out and start a tutoring business?

I know the idea of a nursing student tutor doesn't sound profitable, but it can be. It just all depends on the way you market your services and what you offer. As an educator to the new nursing generation, you can branch out and offer other services besides strictly nursing school tutoring.

The possibilities are numerous. Think about offering courses on how to effectively study in general. You can specialize by adding courses on the HESI, NCLEX, and even certifications beyond nursing school like the CCRN or CEN.

Once again, like an NCLEX review instructor, these courses can be carried out online or in person. And, you can still set up 1-on-1 tutoring sessions for extra cash. You may even consider meeting with local schools to speak with them about potential referrals during the school year.

Materials needed to start your own tutoring business would vary depending on what services you will be offering. If you want to focus on general studying tips then develop the products needed (study sheets, workbooks, etc). Determine your curriculum and how you plan to carry out your tutoring business.

Additional Resources:
Your Nursing Tutor
http://www.yournursingtutor.com

Potential Start-up costs: $1,000 or less

Additional degree required: No

Sole venture or partnership: Either

Mobile, Online or Brick & Mortar: Any

Potential products to upsell: Your own general study materials, offering 1-on-1 tutoring, developing other nursing related courses (HESI, NCLEX, CCRN, etc.)

BLS and ACLS Instructor

In my nursing experience, I have known a few nurses who are certified BLS or ACLS instructors, but they did not take advantage of their situation. They would teach a class occasionally for the extra money; but for some reason, they wouldn't pursue it from a business standpoint.

As a BLS/ACLS instructor, you will need equipment and a place to hold the course, but this can easily be worked out for a business venture. I know a couple who rents an apartment as their office and classrooms. You could also pursue this business on a mobile basis. I could see dedicating an SUV or van to storing and transporting the equipment to locations convenient to those needing to take a class.

This business could be quite profitable when you take into consideration that the average ACLS class costs around $200. If you add in BLS, you could charge at least $250 per student. I'm sure you're thinking about the costs associated with the necessary equipment—which can be costly, but don't fret. The costs aren't recurring, meaning that once you get set up with what you need you won't need to buy new equipment on a regular basis.

The equipment list would include but is not limited to: mannequins, AED, crash cart, TV and DVD player, and The American Heart Association books and guides. As you can see many of the big-ticket items don't need to be replaced on a yearly basis.

Additional Resources:
http://www.gaebler.com/How-to-Start-a-CPR-Instruction-School.htm

Potential Start-up costs: $5,000+

Additional degree required: No

Sole venture or partnership: Either

Mobile, Online, or Brick & Mortar: Mobile or Brick & Mortar

Potential products to upsell: Selling AEDs to companies and individuals, charging extra for mobile services

Educational Vacation Seminars

Are you well-versed in a particular subject matter that could help other nurses? Can what you know be applied to continuing education hours for nurses? Do you like to travel? If you answered yes to all of the above, why not use your expertise to host seminars in desirable travel locations?

If I had a choice between going to a seminar in my backyard at the local Marriot or on a Hawaiian cruise, I'd choose the cruise hands down because I'd get to learn and vacation at the same time.

This venture could be handled on your own, but I'd want to incorporate a partner for the sheer size of each seminar. You would have to find a desirable travel destination and work out an arrangement with a venue to host your seminar. This could potentially include a hotel, cruise ship or cozy bed and breakfast retreat-style venue.

In addition, you have to market your services well, because an educational vacation with just one participant is: 1) Not worth the time and hassle it took to put the seminar together and 2) No fun at all!

Additional Resources: See examples at:
http://www.travelmedicalseminars.com/

http://www.continuingeducation.net/

Potential Start-up costs: $2,000

Additional degree required: No

Sole venture or partnership: Sole, but I would suggest a partnership

Mobile, Online, or Brick & Mortar: Mobile

Potential products to upsell: Books and other educational materials, consultation services, bags, mugs, pens and pencils with your logo.

Medical Spanish for Healthcare Providers Instructor

Are you a bilingual nurse? Being bilingual in certain areas can pay off handsomely for healthcare providers who are well versed in Spanish or any other regional foreign language for the area.

This business would be an easy set-up for someone fluent in multiple languages. I would start out by making educational materials consisting of the most common phrases used in the healthcare setting. I, for one, would love to be able to carry out a full assessment in Spanish. You could start with basic questions and answers.

You could offer your services to tutor local nurses one-on-one or even contract out a 4-6 week class with a hospital who wants to invest in more nurses becoming bilingual and decreasing the cost of medical interpreters. This could be a very lucrative career for the right person.

Additional Resources: Medical Spanish.com: http://www.medicalspanish.com
My Spanish Teacher:
http://www.myspanishteacher.com

Potential Start-up costs: $500 or less

Additional degree required: No

Sole venture or partnership: Sole

Mobile, Online, or Brick & Mortar: Mobile

Potential products to upsell: Online course, books, pocket-guide for most commonly used terms and phrases.

CE Online Bank or Registry

Many states now require nurses to have a certain number of continuing education credits each year before renewing their license. Continuing education credits can be completed in an online format or in-person. A great idea for a nurse in education or is computer savvy can set up an online CEU bank for nurses and other healthcare professionals.

Charge based on the type of CEUs and the number of CEUs per course. You could charge a one-time yearly (or monthly) fee and let individuals take all the CEUs they need during the specified period. To start this type of business you would have to have a website with a large bank of CEUs and a shopping cart on the site set up.

Additional Resources:
http://nursece4less.com

Potential Start-up costs: $500 or less

Additional degree required: No

Sole venture or partnership: Sole

Mobile, Online, or Brick & Mortar: Mobile

Potential products to upsell: Courses from other CE providers (arrange affiliate commissions from those online sites).

ESL instructor

This business idea is good for someone who has a good command of the English language and likes to teach. It's not necessarily nursing related per say, but you could easily set yourself up as a teacher for ESL.

Certifications are required in most states to become an ESL instructor. If you're interested in this type of business, research your state's requirement for instructors. Once you obtain your ESL certification, you could approach the business in one of two ways: online or in person.

An online set-up would take more work in the beginning while setting up videos and courses, but later you have to ability to make money even while you sleep, and that's always a good thing! Teaching in person wouldn't need much money to start because you could go to local community centers in neighborhoods that have many people who aren't English speakers. Ask to rent out a room on a weekly or monthly basis for your classes.

Additional Resources:
https://certificationmap.com/faq/esl-certification

Potential Start-up costs: $300+

Additional degree required: Yes, ESL certification

Sole venture or partnership: Sole

Mobile, Online, or Brick & Mortar: Online or Brick & Mortar

Potential products or services to upsell:

Nurse Consultant

Out of all the careers listed in this book, the nurse consultant must be the most versatile. A whole book can be written about the nurse consultant, but I'm going to attempt to give you an overview of this adaptable business venture and limit it to a few pages. The true definition of a consultant is "one who gives professional advice or services in a particular area." This is a pretty broad definition, but one which could fit a nurse well.

Unlike other professional jobs, the nurse consultant does not need any more education than the diploma you received from nursing school. As a nurse consultant, your special expertise is whatever you do best. Take me for instance. My coworkers were always approaching me, asking what they should do with their careers. Over the years, I've given so much advice about nursing careers and education, I figured I could start a business doing the same thing and extend my reach beyond my coworkers.

I am in fact a nursing career consultant. That's what ReNursing Career Consulting is all about.

You can become a consultant in any area where you have a passion or expertise. I've heard of people who label themselves as sleep consultants for children—and they're not even nurses! They are just your normal run-of-the-mill moms who saw a need and filled it. Can you imagine if an L&D nurse who was also a mom started a business like that? That would be perfect and she would be creditable--if I had the choice of seeing someone who was just a mom (no bashing here, moms!) vs. someone who was a mom and L&D nurse, I would automatically choose the nurse.

Any nursing specialty you have can be translated into a nurse consultant business. My background includes working in the ICU for the last 8 years. Since I've been around awhile, I've seen systems that work well and systems that don't. If I were not a career consultant, I would seriously consider working as a consultant who helps streamline the nursing workplace to help reduce stress and burnout. I don' know what to call this type of consultant, but I bet if I brainstormed long enough and found a hospital system who cared about nursing turnover, I could make a pretty good business out of it.

The equipment list you need to start your consulting business is slim: a typical home office, business cards, and a website. You may need a few specific items depending on what type of consultant you aspire to be.

Additional Resources: www.renursing.com

Potential Start-up costs: $500 or less

Additional degree required: No

Sole venture or partnership: Either

Mobile, Online, or Brick & Mortar: Online or Brick & Mortar

Potential products to upsell: Books, seminars, courses

Other potential Nurse Consultant businesses:
Newborn Nurse Consultant
This type of consulting would consist of helping new parents transition into their new role. Newborns don't come with instruction manuals, and a consultant could help fill in that void. Do you have any special hacks that could help new parents adjust to life with a new baby, things like getting the baby on a feeding schedule? If you do, I'm sure many new parents would be willing to pay.

Sleep Nurse Consultant
A Sleep Nurse Consultant is just that, a sleep consultant for small children. The Sleep Nurse

Consultant would ideally work with infants to pre-school aged children. This job would require some overnights at the child's home to determine exactly what the problem is and time to remedy the problem. Some consulting may be done remotely, but remember if you do on-site consulting you can charge extra for your time because it is an overnight shift.

Social Media Consultant
A Social Media Consultant isn't really nursing related, but you can definitely market your services to a healthcare related entity! If you're seriously social media savvy with all the major social media sites (i.e., Facebook, Twitter, Instagram, Pinterest, etc.) then market your services and get paid for it! A Social Media Consultant would keep up with all social media accounts associated with a particular business to market for the company and also interact with customers virtually.

Nursing Career Consultant
Like I mentioned earlier, a Nursing Career Consultant will help guide other nurses into a career path that suits them. The range of services are also broad and involve phone or in-person consulting, teaching classes, writing

books and reviewing and writing resumes for nurses.

Legal Nurse Consultant

The purpose of a legal nurse consultant is to help legal professionals to understand the terminology and procedures used in the medical profession. They often work in support of attorneys during malpractice lawsuits, medical fraud cases, or criminal conduct requiring medical insight. They are involved in personal injury cases, worker's compensation cases, and toxic torts.

You can find more information about these duties at http://everynurse.org/becoming-a-legal-nurse-consultant/

Fitness Nurse Consultant

I once had a fellow colleague who sold a popular nutritional supplement while he worked as a nurse. This guy was also really buff and you could tell he worked out. It was easy to buy supplements from him since you believed if they made him look so good, they would work for you too. After further conversation with him, I realized he did personal training on the side as well. After even further conversation, I found out he had a Kinesiology degree before he went on to nursing! I told him, "Do you realize with your credentials you could easily market yourself as a Fitness Nurse Consultant and make a significant income doing so?"

He could easily integrate selling supplements, personal training, and his nursing and kinesiology degrees to make a very profitable business.

Survey Nurse Consultant
Do you have a prior career in nursing doing state surveys for facilities? If so, why not hire yourself out as an independent contractor and make a business out of it? Market yourself to those who have had a record of violations or not doing well on inspections and offer to go in and straighten out their issues...for a fee of course.

My point is, dear nurses, capitalize off what you know!

Chapter 4
Child Services Businesses

After-hours Daycare

Nurses are known for working odd hours- 8hrs, 12hrs, 16hrs, days, evenings, nights and weekends. Those with kids sometimes have a difficult time finding childcare that correlates with their schedule. Opening an after-hours daycare in the right area could be a lucrative business.

I see this daycare having overnight hours for parents who work the graveyard shift. The daycare would be open on weekends too, since that is a hard time to find a babysitter as well. You target parents are those who do not work traditional 9-5 jobs and work weekends. This is a very specific niche market and this means money.

You could charge for full-time care, part-time care, and offer drop-in rates for someone needing a babysitter at the last minute. Because your daycare is open odd hours, you could easily charge more than average rates. I am sure parents would gladly pay if they had no one else to watch the kids.

There are many start-up costs involved in opening a daycare. As a daycare owner, you have to have a building for the daycare; this can be a home or a commercial location. Each state has specific rules on how a daycare is set up, regulated, and licensed.

Things to consider when opening a daycare center include; attending classes required by the state to obtain licensing, background checks, hiring employees, specific equipment for the daycare (high chairs, cots, cribs, fire extinguishers, etc.) and getting liability insurance.

Starting a daycare is tedious and costly, but well worth it if you have a passion for children and want to start a business.

Additional Resources:
http://www.nursesfordaycare.com

Potential Start-up costs: $10,000+

Additional degree required: No

Sole venture or partnership: Partnership

Mobile, Online, or Brick & Mortar: Brick & Mortar

Potential products to upsell: T-shirts and other items with your company logo, host an event (art night, pajama party for the local community), courses to promote child safety

Mobile School Nurse

Many school districts have felt the pain of budget cuts during recent years. Often, they have tried to preserve their teaching positions but have eliminated staff jobs like the school nurse. It seemed like they had no other choice.

You can give them the answer to their troubles by providing a service that has nurses rotating through the different schools, and/or providing on-scene minor emergency services. The schools would be able to pay well because they would not have to cover healthcare or retirement benefits. You wouldn't either unless the business explodes with growth. In those cases, you could probably set up another company for additional school districts.

Your service can take advantage of the availability of many nurses who are off-shift for much of the week. All that would be needed is a basic kit of common medical supplies like bandages, antiseptics, EpiPens, hot/cold compresses, etc. Nurses could use their own cars for the transportation (with a mileage allowance). Pediatric nurses would be especially great in this business.

Startup costs would be quickly recovered. Income would be stable and based on a contract agreement.

Additional Resources:
An example from Chicago -
http://catalyst-chicago.org/2015/06/30-million-contract-to-privatize-certified-school-nurses/

Potential Start-up costs: $1,000 or less

Additional degree required: None

Sole venture or partnership: Sole

Mobile, Online or Brick & Mortar: Mobile

Potential products to upsell:
Vaccination programs, health education.

In-hospital Daycare Center

This version of a daycare is golden, and I would invest in it if I weren't neck deep in my own business endeavors right now. How many people have to lose work because their childcare fell through? Numerous. How many hospitals struggle with staff retention or short staffing because of their employees having childcare issues? Many.

For this daycare set up, it would require an individual to set one up in the hospital. Many hospitals have empty rooms or wings for that matter that can be converted into a daycare center for children of the employees. I would approach a hospital and ask to rent an unused space for the center. In addition, tell the hospital you will give them a percent of profits for each child enrolled in the center.

You will win because you will never run out of clientele since your center is located where hundreds and sometimes thousands of people work each day. The hospital will win because they will have greater employee satisfaction, fewer call-ins, and increased productivity, not to mention an additional profit if you choose to go this route.

Additional Resources:
http://www.nursesfordaycare.com

Potential Start-up costs: $50,000+

Additional degree required: No

Sole venture or partnership: Partnership

Mobile, Online, or Brick & Mortar: Brick & Mortar

Potential products to upsell: FRANCHISE!

Sick Daycare Center

A spin on the traditional daycare is the sick daycare center. Parents lose many workdays when they have to stay home with a sick child because their regular daycare will not take them because of illness. It's an absolute requirement to have a nurse on staff to assess the ill child and monitor their progress while under their care.

This daycare model uses more of the nurses' expertise although the concept is pretty much the same. A sick daycare center can be modeled one of two ways: (1) a daycare who only cares for sick children or (2) a "sick bay" housed within a regular center.

Although equipped to care for sick children, there must be guidelines in place for which types of illnesses are allowed and what types of illnesses are not. Typically, highly infectious diseases such as chicken pox, high fever, and infectious diarrhea would not be permitted in this scenario.

Additional Resources:
http://www.nursesfordaycare.com

Potential Start-up costs: $10,000+

Additional degree required: No

Sole venture or partnership: Partnership

Mobile, Online, or Brick & Mortar: Brick & Mortar

Potential products to upsell: T-shirts and other items with your company logo, host an event (art night, pajama party for the local community), courses to promote child safety.

Nanny Referral Agency

Do you love children, but you don't necessarily want to work directly with them as a caregiver? Consider starting a Nanny Placement agency for busy parents who don't have time to vet a proper caregiver for their child.

As a Nanny referral agency, you will take the time to properly screen potential nannies and babysitters for families that need childcare outside of a daycare setting. Agencies do the major legwork such as drug screens, references, and making sure the candidate has CPR and any other basic childcare certifications needed.

You can work your Nanny Referral agency out of the comfort of your own home, although I would strongly recommend meeting all candidates face-to-face in a public place. If you are a parent, I would even bring your own child along as a test – just to see how the caregiver interacts with children.

Start up costs for this type of venture would be on the lower end if you're starting out on your own, but well into the thousands if you purchase a Nanny referral franchise. For the sake of the book, let's just say you are doing this on your own. You would need a computer with Internet access, liability insurance for your company and subscriptions for the companies doing the actual background and criminal checks.

Additional Resources:
Association of Premier Nanny Agencies
http://www.theapna.org
International Nanny Association:
http://www.nanny.org

Potential Start-up costs: $2,000+

Additional degree required: No

Sole venture or partnership: Sole

Mobile, Online, or Brick & Mortar: Online

Potential products to upsell: T-shirts and other items with your company logo, host an event (art night, pajama party for the local community), courses to promote child safety.

Adoption Escort Services

This is another potential business venture that would serve a neonatal or pediatric nurse well. Offering Adoption Escort services to parents going though the adoption process would be of great benefit during a very stressful, otherwise joyous, time in their lives.

As an Adoption Escort, you would travel with the parents to their child's home of origin (domestic or international) and bring them back to their new home. During this time you will help with travel issues of getting through customs, offer general childcare and guidance during the first few days, and be an extra-set of hands during the traveling process.

Your travel and accommodations, in addition to your services, are where you will make your money.

Additional Resources: Sky Nurses – http://www.skynurses.com

Potential Start-up costs: $1,000 +

Additional degree required: No

Sole venture or partnership: Either

Mobile, Online, or Brick & Mortar: Mobile

Potential products to upsell: Franchise opportunity

Home Safety Assessment Nurse

Here's another business that involves children, but not in a typical way. Expectant parents often worry about baby-proofing their home to make it safe for their new addition. Read up on different baby proofing safety measures and offer to childproof a home for a fee.

This is a hands-on business, but you could also host safety classes at local community centers for a fee. You could also provide basic home safety assessment visits, just to point out any obvious safety concerns in the home and allow the parents to baby proof on their own.

Another potential source of income could be becoming a distributor of the safety products you use. You'd have to contact each company and ask if you would get a commission for selling their devices.

Additional Resources:
https://www.ncoa.org/wp-content/uploads/Creative_Practices-Home_Safety_Report.pdf

http://mhcc.maryland.gov/consumerinfo/longtermcare/HomeSafetyAssessment.aspx

Potential Start-up costs: $100

Additional degree required: None

Sole venture or partnership: Sole

Mobile, Online, or Brick & Mortar: Mobile

Potential products or services to upsell: Childproofing equipment, consulting services.

Chapter 5
Skills Businesses

Foot Care Nurse

If you have an interest in feet and helping the elderly and diabetic population, this could be the business opportunity for you. A foot-care nurse helps patients who are unable to properly care for their feet.

Services a foot care nurse can provide include; foot and nail assessment, shoe wear assessment, corn and callus care, nail debridement, wound assessment and more. Some providers can bill Medicare or offer cash only services.

As a foot-care nurse you can work out of your own home, the patients home, long-term care facilities, or nursing homes. You can work out a deal with the local nursing home by offering to come to their facility on a monthly basis or you can contract your services out privately.

Additional Resources:

American Foot Care Nurses Association: http://www.afcna.org
Foot Care Nurses, LLC:
http://www.footcarenursesllc.com

Potential Start-up costs: $1,000 or less

Additional degree required: No

Sole venture or partnership: Solo

Mobile, Online, or Brick & Mortar: Mobile

Potential products to upsell: Homemade creams and lotions, Pedi-eggs, files, nail clippers with your logo, online educational course.

PICC/Midline Insertion Nurse

Many nurses have learned how to insert PICC's or Midlines on the job and insert these lines within their own hospital setting, but did you ever think of taking it out of the hospital and doing it on your own?

PICC/Midline nurses have a valuable skill that they can use to make a profitable business out of. You would need a working relationship with the suppliers of the insertion kits and facilities you would market to. In addition, you'd need to have a relationship with an x-ray service if you plan to insert lines in a home health setting to verify placement.

These services could be done on a cash pay basis in Skilled Nursing Facilities (SNF's), nursing homes, and patients needing home health services. Some outside PICC nurses charge $150 per line placement. PICC lines do require routine maintenance by a nurse as well.

Start-up costs would include insertion kits, a portable ultrasound, flushes, and caps for the injection ports.

Additional Resources:
http://piccresource.com/piccnurseblog/picc-certification-what-does-it-mean/

Potential Start-up costs: $10,000+ depending on ultrasound equipment purchased

Additional degree required: No

Sole venture or partnership: Sole

Mobile, Online, or Brick & Mortar: Mobile

Potential products to upsell: Educational materials related to vascular access, training for others who would like to insert PICCs/Midlines

EKG Instructor

Are you good at reading EKG's? Do your co-workers always come to you for assistance reading your strips? Consider starting a business teaching others the ins and outs of everything EKG.

This business can easily be done in your spare time on your days off. Get copies of strips from the most basic Normal Sinus Rhythm to the most complex Wolf-Parkinson-White syndrome, upload them to your website and give step-by-step details on how to interpret them. This can be in the format of an audio podcast, an online interactive course or simply by presenting a rhythm strip of the day type of post.

Additional Resources:
American Board of Cardiovascular Medicine's (ABCM) Board Certification
http://www.abcmcertification.com/ekg-instructor-board-exams.html

Potential Start-up costs: <$100

Additional degree required: None

Sole venture or partnership: Sole

Mobile, Online, or Brick & Mortar: Online

Potential products to upsell: Calipers, online courses

CNA School

If you enjoy teaching others' this may be the business for you. Just as there is a nursing shortage, many nurses' would agree that there is a nursing aide shortage. I've worked countless times without nurses' aides or with nurses' aides who were (excuse my bluntness) not worth their weight in dirt.

As a CNA school instructor, you would be able to directly influence the future nurses' aides (and potential future nurses) on proper nursing skills. This business venture is going to need a physical building for a skills lab to properly educate your students. You will also need to have computers set-up for your students to take their exit exam from the program.

You would need to check with your state's board of nursing for specific rules and regulations for a CNA school. Start-up costs for this business include rent on a physical property, equipment for a skills lab, books and other educational materials for your students and insurance for your business.

Additional Resources:
CNA Instructor Certification
http://study.com/articles/How_to_Become_a_CNA_Instructor.html

Potential Start-up costs: $10,000 minimum

Additional degree required: No

Sole venture or partnership: Sole

Mobile, Online, or Brick & Mortar: Brick & Mortar

Potential products to upsell: Educational materials related to nurses aide training, training for others who would like to start a CNA school

Skills Training Workshop

If you are exceptionally good at something, say a skill, why not take your expertise on the road and hold training and workshops in different areas of the country? I went to an NP skills workshop and the owner was an NP who was good at several skills and decided to start her own business.

They fly out from their home and host skills workshops at different venues all across the country. It is a great idea, but it will take a lot to put this type of business together. The start-up fees would be high, but you would be able to charge a good price for students who want to attend your workshops.

You would need to get equipment for the types of skills you plan to teach, prepare PowerPoint presentations, submit your workshop agenda to the appropriate board for continuing education, and establish contracts with the venue you'd be holding the workshops in.

Additional Resources:
Top 11 Skills for Successful RN - http://www.topregisterednurse.com/registered-nurse-skills/

Potential Start-up costs: Varies according to the skill being taught and equipment needed.

Additional degree required: No

Sole venture or partnership: Either

Mobile, Online, or Brick & Mortar: Mobile

Potential products or services to upsell: Other courses, either in person or online.

Phlebotomy School

As a nurse, you already learned phlebotomy skills while in school and gained experience on the job. Phlebotomy skills are needed by those who actually want to draw blood on people for a living, so why not open a phlebotomy school? In addition, you could offer refresher courses to those who have been out of practice for a while.

The set-up for this type of school is going to be similar to opening a CNA school. You will need to research your state's rules and regulations to be in compliance in your area. Start-up costs for this business include rent on a physical property, equipment for a skills lab, books and other educational materials for your students and insurance for your business (and students).

Additional Resources:
http://medical2.com/programs/program/certification-workshops

Potential Start-up costs: $10,000 minimum

Additional degree required: No

Sole venture or partnership: Sole

Mobile, Online, or Brick & Mortar: Brick & Mortar

Potential products to upsell: Include basic ECG Certification, CNA certification training, etc.

Chapter 6
Travel Businesses

Vacation Companion Travel Nurse Agency

A Vacation Companion Travel Nurse agency is just what it means – a nurse who travels with an otherwise homebound person while on vacation. There are many variations to this type of business. You can employ only nurses to accompany patients, or you can employ nurses and nurses aides. In addition to nursing care, you can offer general travel services to your clients.

Services a Vacation Companion Travel Nurse would provide are include, but are not limited to; assisting with getting through customs, seating, and care while on the plane or in the car, assistance with loading luggage, administering medications and nursing assistance when at the vacation destination. For this service, your airline tickets, accommodations, and sometimes meals are covered in addition to charging for the actual nursing services.

This business venture will require a significant amount of capital if you want a full-fledged agency with additional staff beside yourself. As an independent contractor, you could offer your traveling services easily. The only issue I see with increased start-up costs as an independent contractor is being licensed in the states where you intend to travel. If you were to travel to a state that did not recognize your license, you would be in violation of the law to offer nursing services there. A state that recognizes compact licensure would make this somewhat easier and less costly for someone who wants to pursue this type of business.

Additional Resources:
Trip Nurse- http://www.tripnurse.com
Commercial Medical *Escorts-*
http://www.commercialmedicalescorts.com
Sky Nurses- http://www.skynurses.com

Potential Start-up costs: $1,000 +

Additional degree required: None, but additional state licensure may be required depending on where you plan to travel.

Sole venture or partnership: Either

Mobile, Online, or Brick & Mortar: Mobile

Potential products to upsell: Travel agency services, travel insurance, home visits by an MD or NP

Medical Transport

If you don't mind flying and being on-call for travel consider starting a medical transportation business. Many wealthy people with health concerns need to travel outside their homes or hospitals for one reason or another.

As a nurse who focuses on medical transportation, you could do ground transportation by taking patients to and from medical facilities or you can hire yourself out as a nurse who does air transportation. These patients are not usually critical enough to use an ambulance for transportation, but just need medical escort.

I think a nurse with a strong background would do just fine in this type of business. Start-up fees for ground transportation would be higher since you would need a van, stretcher, and other transportation-related medical supplies. With the air transportation business, you would just need to market yourself as someone willing to escort patients who needed to travel.

Additional Resources:
http://www.ncsl.org/research/transportation/non-emergency-medical-transportation-a-vital-lifeline-for-a-healthy-community.aspx

Potential Start-up costs: $10,000+ (depending on air or ground transportation)

Additional degree required: None

Sole venture or partnership: Sole or Partnership

Mobile, Online, or Brick & Mortar: Mobile

Potential products to upsell: Consulting services, transport errands.

Mobile Flu Vaccine Clinic

I've actually met a nurse who started a flu vaccine clinic, and it sounded like an interesting business idea. She bought her supplies, hired a few nurses, and set-up shop at local facilities to give flu shots. From what I hear, her business was quite profitable.

This venture could be done on a small-scale basis at first until you land bigger and bigger contracts that require hundreds of injections per clinic. The cost for set-up would be small. You would need a table, a chair, and supplies for the injections. Needles and syringes are inexpensive, and the flu season is limited, so you will not need to keep stock all year round.

An additional optional business is a pet vaccination clinic, though the income potential may be less.

Additional Resources:
For Texas, but similar information applies -
https://www.dshs.texas.gov/immunize/nurse/default.shtm

Potential Start-up costs: $1000+

Additional degree required: None

Sole venture or partnership: Sole

Mobile, Online, or Brick & Mortar: Mobile

Potential products to upsell: Consulting services for others who want to start a mobile vaccine clinic

Mobile Infusion (Hang-Over Clinic)

If the club scene is big in your area, consider opening a mobile hangover clinic to help people sober up after a night of partying. Similar to a food truck van, the van would park in front of certain establishments to give infusions for those coming out of the bar.

A van would be needed along with nurses willing to work with the inebriated population, you may want to include a security guard as staff too just in case things get rowdy.

During the day when pubic intoxication is not at its peak, you can offer your services to gym-rats who want a cocktail of vitamins after a hard workout. You can even consider setting up at the finish line of a race for runners who may be in need of hydration after running a marathon.

Additional Resources:
Examples from two states -
http://pushlv.com/

http://ivtherapyhouston.com/hangover/

Potential Start-up costs: $10,000+

Additional degree required: None

Sole venture or partnership: Partnership

Mobile, Online, or Brick & Mortar: Mobile

Potential products to upsell: Supplements.

Public Speaker

If you have ever been told you have a knack for speaking and making others feel good, maybe you should consider being a public speaker. Use your experience as a nurse to travel to different venues giving speeches around your topic of expertise.

The start-up costs for this type of business are relatively low, but like any other business, you will have to market your services. Why exactly would someone want to hire you as a speaker? In order for this to be a profitable business, you have to brand yourself with your particular expertise. You're going to have to identify an audience before people will want to book you for events. How you go about this is left to your own devices and can be accomplished in many ways.

You may also want to train other medical professionals to improve their communication skills. (http://successfully-speaking.com/medical-professionals/

Additional Resources:
Find public speaking opportunities -
http://famousinyourfield.com/17-ways-to-find-speaking-opportunities/

Potential Start-up costs: $100

Additional degree required: None

Sole venture or partnership: Sole

Mobile, Online, or Brick & Mortar: Mobile

Potential products to upsell: Consulting Services for others wanting to be a public speaker, books.

Chapter 7
Tech Savvy Businesses

Website or Domain Flipper

Ever heard of house flipping where you buy a run-down home, put a little TLC into it and then re-sell it for a higher profit? That takes a lot of time, money, and hard work. But, there is another form of flipping that would work well with the nurse who is skilled with developing Internet websites.

Enter in the world of website or domain flipping. Website flipping involves taking an established website with good traffic flow (actual or potential) and selling it to another for a profit. This is a website you could already own (like my website www.renursing.com) or a website you brought specifically with the intention of sprucing it up a bit and selling.

Websites and domains can command anywhere from a few hundred up into the thousands. Unlike house flipping, you do not need tons of capital to get started either. This is something that can easily be worked around a nurse's schedule to make extra cash. I don't know the full-fledged business potential, but profits could surely get you extra income to put into other bigger business ventures.

Additional Resources:
Flippa: http://www.flippa.com,
Valuate: http://www.valuate.com,

Potential Start-up costs: $500 or less depending on the type of site or domain you purchase

Additional degree required: No

Sole venture or partnership: Sole

Mobile, Online or Brick & Mortar: Online

Potential products to upsell: Website coding services, SEO services, copywriting for websites.

Medical Website Designer

If you are tech savvy and know how to design websites, then why not use your skill to be a Medical Website Designer? You can use your background as a nurse to advertise to a specific niche market or you can design websites for the masses.

Many start-ups need websites. Most try to do them on their own and when finished, they look unprofessional. An unprofessional website will do nothing for a business.

The beauty of being a Medical Website Designer is that you can work strictly from home and get paid a pretty good price per website you complete.

Additional Resources:
Web Design Training -
http://www.creativebloq.com/web-design/training-online-resources-812225

Free & Cheap Online Courses
https://www.udemy.com/courses/search/?q=web design&src=ukw&lang=en

Potential Start-up costs: <$1,000

Additional degree required: No

Sole venture or partnership: Sole

Mobile, Online, or Brick & Mortar: Online

Potential products to upsell: Copywriting for websites, setting up social media account pages (Twitter, Facebook, Instagram, etc)

App Developer

Do you have a great idea for an app? Why not get in gear and get it developed to sell to the masses?

New apps pop up every day, but the right app could make you a lot of money. Health and wellness is a big sector now and combined with technology it could make for a great business idea. Your app could be anything- something that could help nurses out every day or even the general population.

Unless you have programming skills, this is a job you'd have to hire out. If you do decide to build an app make sure you make it both Apple and Android compatible.

Additional Resources:
https://www.udemy.com/courses/search/?q=app%20development&src=ukw&lang=en

Potential Start-up costs: $500+

Additional degree required: None

Sole venture or partnership: Sole

Mobile, Online, or Brick & Mortar: Online

Potential products or services to upsell: Courses on app development, Consulting on how to start an app developer business

Podcaster

If you don't like blogging but have a lot of information to share, why not try your hand at starting a podcast series? To get started with a podcasting, you would first need a website and a large enough following to eventually make money.

The money may not come directly from your podcasts, but the podcasts themselves could turn into courses, public speaking events, and consulting for the topic you focus on.

Podcasting is relatively easy to get into, so I hear. The basic set-up is a computer with a good quality microphone for sound quality, software for audio recording, and a place to host your podcasts (your site or a podcast hosting service).

Additional Resources:
Courses -
https://www.udemy.com/courses/search/?q=podcasting&src=ukw&lang=en

Potential Start-up costs: $500+

Additional degree required: None

Sole venture or partnership: Sole

Mobile, Online, or Brick & Mortar: Online

Potential products or services to upsell: Courses on domain flipping, books.

Chapter 8
Health and Wellness Businesses

Health and Wellness Spa

A health and wellness spa would be an excellent opportunity for a nurse who has a cosmetic or plastic surgery background. These types of clinics are popping up everywhere because everyone wants to be beautiful. If you offer services such as Botox, Restalyne, and other cosmetic procedures, you would have a growing client base without much hassle in finding patients. The best part of this type of business? It's a cash-only practice!

You'd need a good retail or medical space to locate your clinic in addition to deciding what kind of procedures you want to perform in your clinic. If you are an LPN or RN (or even an NP in some states) you will need to add a physician collaborator for the clinic to your payroll. In addition to your physical staffing needs, you will need to purchase your equipment needed for the procedures you'll be performing.

Additional Resources:
What you should know before…
http://www.massagetoday.com/mpacms/mt/article.php?id=13358

How to Start Your Own Day Spa
http://smallbusiness.chron.com/start-own-day-spa-business-4813.html

Health and Wellness Coach -
https://www.udemy.com/courses/search/?q=health and wellness coach&src=sac&kw=health and wellness spa&lang=en

Potential Start-up costs: $10,000 minimum

Additional degree required: No

Sole venture or partnership: Sole

Mobile, Online, or Brick & Mortar: Brick & Mortar

Potential products to upsell:
Lotions and skincare products, nutritional supplements.

Fitness studio

This type of business is good for the nurse who has a lot of capital to invest and lives fitness. Boutique fitness studios are all the rage and cover every fitness fad imaginable from Pilates, yoga, to rowing and everything in between. Big profits can be made if you keep your fitness classes engaging and fun so people will want to come back. Boutique studios are charging up to $250 per month for memberships!

Include another value-based service like nutritional counseling or prenatal classes, and you'll keep your customers coming back for more. Word of mouth is big in this type of industry so you'll have to keep up with your social media accounts to get people pumped up to workout in your studio.

With this type of venture, unless you have enough money to pay many employees you're going to have to quit your day job as a nurse to manage the business and make sure your clients get the boutique experience they want.

Additional Resources:
http://www.shape.com/lifestyle/mind-and-body/beginner-s-guide-starting-your-own-fitness-studio

Potential Start-up costs: $100,000+

Additional degree required: None

Sole venture or partnership: Either

Mobile, Online or Brick & Mortar: Brick & mortar

Additional products or services to upsell: T-shirts, personal training sessions

Pre/intra/post-natal fitness instructor

Getting and staying healthy is a big business, especially when you're expecting or have just had a baby. Market a business specifically for pregnant women who want to have a healthy pregnancy and control their weight gain during pregnancy. For those who have just had babies offer gentle exercises after they are cleared from their doctor.

This is a special population and I'm sure that a Labor and Delivery or Mom and Baby nurse would make a great instructor to these moms. This business can take on a multitude of forms by offering online courses, in-home training, or opening a specialized facility.

Additional Resources:
Pre and Post-natal Fitness Certification -
http://store.afpafitness.com/pre-and-post-natal-fitness-specialist-certification/

Oh Baby Training
https://www.ohbabyfitness.com/pre-postnatal-fitness-training

Potential Start-up costs: $1000+ (depending on business model)

Additional degree required: None

Sole venture or partnership: Sole

Mobile, Online or Brick & Mortar: Any

Potential products or services to Up-sell: Exercise equipment, yoga mats, nutritional and skin care supplements.

Nachole Johnson

Massage Nurse

Let's face it… nurses' have a tough job. The work can be backbreaking- day in and day out. Who wouldn't like a massage after a hard day's work? I don't know of anyone who would turn that offer down!

How about starting a nursing massage business? There are many business models this could work under. The focus could be on nurses only offering on-site massages to local hospitals at the beginning of each major shift. You could even contract out your services to other non-healthcare related businesses for different events. Another option is contracting with a local orthopedic or sports medicine doctor to provide massages for their patients. Or you could focus on the general public in your own massage studio.

This business model can be started and run by a sole person or you could even add a partner and the model would still work well. There are also potential products you could offer to increase your profits. You could offer aromatherapy and other relaxing materials for purchase when massaging your clients.

You do need to be licensed as a massage therapist in order to pursue this entrepreneurial venture. There are many schools across the country that provide this type of training. Tuition varies for each program, but if this is something you want to do make it happen!

Additional Resources:
American Massage Therapy Association
http://www.amtamassage.org
Massage Association & Liability Insurance for Massage Professionals http://www.abmp.com
National Association of Massage Therapists
http://www.namtonline.com

Potential Start-up costs: $1,000 and up (not including education & licensing)

Additional degree required: Yes

Sole venture or partnership: Either

Mobile, Online or Brick & Mortar: Either mobile or brick or mortar

Potential products to upsell: Aromathcrapy, candles, relaxing music CD's

Chapter 9
Care-giving Businesses

Patient Advocate

Have you ever taken care of a patient who just doesn't have a clue about their own medical care? Many patients don't know why they are on certain medications and what their medical conditions are. I cringe when I come across a patient uninformed about their own care.

As a nurse, you can help patients like this and become a patient advocate. A patient advocate helps patients with the lingo of healthcare by attending doctors appointments with them and educating them on their condition. They can help coordinate appointments, educated on medications and administration, and even help with insurance queries.

This is a career that is best served with an experienced nurse and you can specialize in your current area of expertise (cardiology, geriatrics, pediatrics, etc).

Additional Resources: RN Patient Advocates
http://www.patientadvocates.com
Alliance of Professional Health Advocates
http://www.aphadvocates.org

Potential Start-up costs: <$1,000

Additional degree required: No

Sole venture or partnership: Sole

Mobile, Online, or Brick & Mortar: Mobile

Potential products to upsell: Books, courses, consulting, ad space on site, web developer business.

Case Manager

Many of you may have experience as a case manager at your job. Why not branch out on your own? Case managers coordinate care for patients that may have complex needs after a hospitalization or injury. This includes discharge planning and reviewing medical records to ensure patients are receiving the best care possible.

This is another low-cost entry business if you have the skills and tenacity to market yourself. Consider marketing yourself to smaller establishments who may not have a dedicated case manager on site.

Additional Resources:
https://ccmcertification.org/case-managers/board-certified-case-manager

https://www.acmaweb.org/acm/

Potential Start-up costs: $500

Additional degree required: None

Sole venture or partnership: Sole

Mobile, Online, or Brick & Mortar: Mobile

Potential products to upsell: Consulting, books.

Group Home Owner

Do you have a passion for helping others out in their time of need? Maybe nursing was more than a career for you and actually a calling. If you enjoy helping others why not consider opening a group home specific to an underserved population?

Group home come in all forms and fashions; homeless shelter, teen pregnancy, unemployed veterans, the possibilities are endless for this type of business. The best part is that this type of business is sure to be approved for government funding as a non-profit.

To get started you would obviously need a place where people can call "home." Maybe you have a rental property you can convert (make sure to look into any commercial property laws in residential homes in your area).

Additional Resources:

http://www.careandcompliance.com/administrator-certification-training/administrator-training/online-continuing-education/group-home-administrators-ceu.html

Potential Start-up costs: $1,000+

Additional degree required: None

Sole venture or partnership: Either

Mobile, Online, or Brick & Mortar: Brick & Mortar

Potential products to upsell: Consulting.

Pet Therapy Service

The sick and elderly tend to love pets. For the most part, when someone encounters a dog or cat (just like a baby) they brighten up. Obviously, when someone is sick and in a hospital setting, they may not get to see animals often-- this is where you come in.

Pet therapy services are usually on a volunteer basis, but it costs money to train and certify animals for therapy. As a pet lover, you can train animals for Pet Therapy services.

Additional Resources:
http://www.therapydogsunited.org

Potential Start-up costs:

Additional degree required: Certification

Sole venture or partnership: Sole or partnership

Mobile, Online, or Brick & Mortar: Mobile or Brick & Mortar

Potential products to upsell: Pet supplies--clothing, leashes, bowls, etc.

Home Health Agency

This type of business is good for the nurse who loves to spend a little more time with their patients and really get to know them. In my time as a Home Visit NP, I really enjoyed talking to my patients and getting to know them when I made my visits. This entrepreneurial venture will take a lot more work (and capital) than other careers in this book, simply because it is a massive undertaking.

A Home Health Agency not only needs you, a nurse, but they also need other disciples in the healthcare industry to be even remotely competitive. You will need to foster relationships with doctors, physical and occupational therapists and home health aides to name a few. Contracts will have to be established with insurance companies, Medicare, Medicaid, and any other state-required accreditation and licenses.

Additional Resources:
healthcarelicensing.com
http://www.healthcarelicensing.com

Potential Start-up costs: $10,000 +

Additional degree required: No

Sole venture or partnership: Either

Mobile, Online, or Brick & Mortar: Mobile

Potential products to upsell: You can partner up with another entrepreneur such as a foot-care nurse to offer to your home health patients. You would take commission off each patient you refer to this individual.

Assisted Living Facility

Instead of having to drive to multiple locations taking care of patients, why not open an Assisted Living facility? An assisted living facility is a home for people who need supervision, but not as much medical care as a nursing home. The assisted living facility houses mainly seniors, but memory care residents as well.

There would be a need for all the amenities of home: a large kitchen and dining area and rooms to house residents. Nursing staff would pass medications and look over the general well being of the residents. There is also typically staff that coordinates activities for the residents like weekly bingo night, field trips, and grocery shopping.

Depending on what facility you will use (personal home or commercial property) the costs for a start-up assisted living facility can vary. If you had spare bedrooms in your home you could open up an assisted living facility (think Bed & Breakfast). As the owner, you may also be able to get government assistance for this type of business.

Long-term care insurance is insurance that some people are taking out for the reason of moving into an assisted living facility in their golden years. To start a facility you would need a large home (think bed & breakfast) or an actual apartment-type building with enough space for common areas such as dining, recreational rooms, and outdoor space.

Some, but not all states, require certification for assisted living managers.

This is a big investment and will likely take a significant loan to get the business up and running. You will need to hire staff from the start; nurses, aides, recreation techs, dietary staff, etc. It is a big undertaking, but with determination, it can be done.

Additional Resources:
Google "Assisted Living Manager" for your state.

Potential Start-up costs: $10,000+

Additional degree required: None

Sole venture or partnership: Partnership

Mobile, Online, or Brick & Mortar: Brick & Mortar

Potential products to upsell: Transportation to doctor appointments, shopping, etc.

Elder Daycare

Here is another caregiving business idea, an elder daycare center. Elder daycares are places the elderly can go for socialization during the day. Some caregivers may want to drop Grandma or Grandpa off for a break just like people do for their children.

In an elder daycare, you wouldn't need residential private space like apartments, but you would need a few rooms for recreation, dining, and just relaxing. This business could be run on drop-in rates or on monthly subscriptions. Schedule plenty of activities during the week to keep the group entertained like bingo, karaoke, and arts and crafts.

Additional Resources:
http://www.caregiverslibrary.org/caregivers-resources/grp-caring-for-yourself/hsgrp-support-systems/what-is-adult-day-care-article.aspx

Potential Start-up costs: 10,000+

Additional degree required: None

Sole venture or partnership: Partnership

Mobile, Online, or Brick & Mortar: Brick & Mortar

Potential products or services to upsell: Day trips, special services like haircuts, laundry services

Chapter 10
Miscellaneous Businesses

Medical Supply Retail Store

As a nurse, you've probably frequented a medical supply retail store a time or two. You have purchased scrubs, jacket, stethoscopes, and scissors when you needed them. If you have always dreamed of having your own retail store, why not open a medical supply store?

This venture is a large undertaking, considering the storefront and the inventory you will need to keep on hand. On the other hand, you could do this strictly online and keep your inventory on hand at home. With the online sales aspect, you will have to deal with shipping and returns of items that do not fit well or just don't work out for some reason or another. Although this is the age of online sales, many people still like shop for their scrubs and accessories in person.

If you decide to go with a retail storefront you will need to invest in a security system since you will have tangible items that can disappear and affect your overall bottom line.

Additional Resources: Check out the medical supply stores within your area, then look at the ones online.

Potential Start-up costs: $10,000+ for storefront, considerably cheaper for online store

Additional degree required: No

Sole venture or partnership: Sole or partnership depending on the model

Mobile, Online, or Brick & Mortar: Online or Brick & Mortar

Potential products to upsell: Scrubs, Jackets, stethoscopes, scissors -anything medical related

Stock Investor

If you are financially well informed, you may be able to make a living from investments.

There's not much to it (or so I've heard). You buy stock, hope it grows, and then sell it for a profit. You can also hold it if you like, but you won't be able to turn a profit until you sell.

There are online investments websites that allow people to start out with as little as $500 to invest. This business venture is a gamble, like any business venture, but you will have to be astute on what kinds of stocks to buy and when to sell. Look at where you spend your money and consider investing in those stocks. I personally own a few based on where I like to spend my money, and they are doing well in the market.

There are numerous resources on this topic, and if done right can yield good income potential. Just be sure to do your homework before you start.

Additional Resources:
Stock Investing Courses -
https://www.udemy.com/courses/search/?q=stock investing&src=ukw&lang=en

Potential Start-up costs: $500 minimum

Additional degree required: No

Sole venture or partnership: Sole

Mobile, Online, or Brick & Mortar: Online

Potential products to upsell: Courses, books, consulting

Real Estate Investor

There are many opportunities in Real Estate that would work well with a nurse's schedule and personality that allow for extra income. Some may think Real Estate is risky, but in the long term, investing in Real Estate proves to be a winner in most cases.

There are dozens of ways to invest in Real Estate such as flipping, buy & hold (rentals), wholesaling, commercial, becoming an agent, etc. The complete list is extensive, but if you want to get into Real Estate and don't know how, there's an avenue for you in this vast field.

A nurses' schedule often allows many days off per week. You can use that time finding, repairing, or selling houses. Out of all careers listed in this book, Real Estate offers the most on education and different avenues to get started in the business.

Additional Resources:
http://www.biggerpockets.com

Courses on Real Estate Investing -
https://www.udemy.com/courses/search/?q=real estate investing&src=sac&kw=real estate&lang=en

Potential Start-up costs: $1,000+ (in most cases)

Additional degree required: No

Sole venture or partnership: Sole or partnership

Mobile, Online, or Brick & Mortar: Mobile

Potential products to upsell: Become a Real Estate agent to earn commission while investing, become a professional home stager for homes on the market.

Inventor

Do you have an awesome idea for a new product that will help others? If so, you could devote your time and energy to becoming a professional inventor.

An invention starts with an idea for a product, a patent, and a working prototype. After those initial three steps are in place, you pitch your product to stores for sales. This is where the tricky part comes into play. If a store likes your product, you want to have enough supply to meet the demand of sales. Therefore, you will need someone to manufacture and distribute your product on a large scale.

On the other hand, if you do get large-scale manufacturing, and your product doesn't do well then you have spent a lot of money and have excess product lying around. Since your idea is a novel one, you will have to market, to get it off the ground.

Make sure you don't skip the patent aspect of a new idea. Although it may be pricey, you don't want someone else stealing your idea and making profits that could have gone in your pocket. Inventing a product involves a lot of time and money, but can be well worth it for the right individual with the right product.

Additional Resources:
Courses on Inventing - https://www.udemy.com/courses/search/?q=inventing&src=sac&kw=inventing&lang=en

Potential Start-up costs: $10,000 minimum

Additional degree required: No

Sole venture or partnership: Sole

Mobile, Online, or Brick & Mortar: Brick & Mortar

Potential products to upsell: Consulting, books.

Franchise

This idea has two options for the business-minded nurse. One is to outright purchase a franchise and the other is to franchise your own existing business idea. Personally, I would go with the second one to keep the most profits, but some may like the idea of a business that is already an established brand. One problem with this model is that you will have to make recurring royalty payments to the franchisor.

Franchise fees vary widely for the type of business you want to start, as do the services you want to offer. There is something for everyone if you want to franchise from house cleaning services, childcare, to restaurants and more. If you want to franchise your own business model you are free to charge what you like as far as initial franchise fees and royalty payments. If seek to franchise your own business, be sure to get a good franchise attorney to draft your contracts.

Additional Resources:
Courses on Franchising -
https://www.udemy.com/courses/search/?q=franchising&src=ukw&lang=en

Potential Start-up costs: $500-$200,000+

Additional degree required: None

Sole venture or partnership: Either

Mobile, Online, or Brick & Mortar: All

Potential products to upsell: Consulting, books.

Crime Scene Clean Up Service

Love CSI or have you ever been intrigued by forensics?

Opening a crime scene cleanup service is a sad and gory, but necessary, service since violent crimes occur every day. I doubt you would have strong competition in this market so that is why I have included it here. Nurses have been known to witness gross things while working and talk about it during lunch without batting an eye.

The start-up for this type of business may be tricky since specialized uniforms and cleaners are needed for bodily fluid cleanup. In addition, you would have to find employees willing to do such dirty work. I imagine the job could get emotionally and physiologically exhausting after time. As a business owner, you would also have to invest in a truck or van to haul your equipment from crime scene to crime scene.

Additional Resources:
Six-figure Income -
http://money.cnn.com/2005/02/28/pf/sixfigs_eleven/

Sample website - http://www.crimeclean-up.com/

Potential Start-up costs: $ 5,000+

Additional degree required: None

Sole venture or partnership: Partnership

Mobile, Online, or Brick & Mortar: Mobile

Potential products to upsell: Hording clean-up services

Nursing Staffing Agency

As a nurse and now a nurse practitioner, I've had my share of working with nurse staffing agencies. They were especially valuable when I wanted to do travel nursing, was in between jobs, or just needed a way to make extra money. I've often wondered if these companies were actually founded by real nurses. Well, even if they weren't this is a field that any nurse can get into.

Who best knows about the business of nursing than a nurse? This business would need an expansive website, so if you're not good at building websites outsource this part of the job.

As the business owner, you would need to find customers on both ends, meaning you need to find employers who need nurses and nurses who need a job and bring them together.

There can be many niches and business models within a staffing agency. You can specialize in a certain nursing specialty like pediatrics or OB. Many different variations can be made based upon you want to focus on. In this type of business, you could be set up like a traditional job board like Indeed or you could run a full-spectrum agency by interviewing nurses and presenting the as candidates to a company looking to hire. Your main issue would be establishing how you would be paid once you find nurses for your clients. Will you charge companies to advertise on your site or will you charge them a set fee after they hire one of your nurses?

Additional Resources:
Google "nursing staff referral service," especially for your state.

Potential Start-up costs: $500+

Additional degree required: None

Sole venture or partnership: Sole

Mobile, Online, or Brick & Mortar: Online

Potential products to upsell: Consulting, books, ad space on site.

Expert Witness Nurse

Here's another business idea for a nurse who is interested in the legal system. As an expert witness, you have to be just that-an expert. Use your years of nursing expertise in the court of law explaining nursing in non-technical language for a jury.

You would need nothing more than your years' of experience and to reach out to local law firms to get your foot in the door. Lawyers may even use you for medical record review if they have a need. The path to becoming an expert witness may not be the easiest business to break into, but it will not break the bank to get in either.

Additional Resources:
https://www.tasanet.com/

Potential Start-up costs: $100

Additional degree required: None

Sole venture or partnership: Sole

Mobile, Online, or Brick & Mortar: Mobile

Potential products to upsell: Consulting, courses.

Subscription Box Service

This is a fun business to start, and I was actually excited enough about the idea that I wanted to start my own subscription box service! Subscription box businesses are big now. Think of any interest or hobby you have and it could be delivered to you home on a monthly basis.

Have you heard of the big subscription box sites like Birch Box, Graze or Bark Box? They all focus on different interests, but they are capitalizing on the beauty of a subscription service.

With a subscription box service, you are getting an ongoing income month-to-month that could go on for many, many months with each customer depending on how much they like your services. Of course, you will have the few customers who try your box for a month and then cancel; but for the most part, subscription box business actually capitalize on hoping people with just forget to cancel their membership. That is wrong, I know, but being in and staying in business involves positive cash flow.

A subscription box service can be done with just about any hobby, career, or interest. If you live in a tourist town, why not consider sending out boxes with different souvenirs each month? Alternatively, if you love peanut butter, start a peanut butter of the month club sending out gourmet jars of peanut butter each month.

This is an awesome idea and I wish I had the time to implement one. You would have to come up with a niche, find vendors, and get your actual subscription box designed. The biggest challenge would be packing and shipping at first, but once you get enough demand you can hire that job out to a distribution center.

Additional Resources:
How to start - https://www.entrepreneur.com/article/244825

Pros and Cons of Running One - http://articles.bplans.com/the-pros-and-cons-of-running-a-subscription-service/

Potential Start-up costs: $500+

Additional degree required: None

Sole venture or partnership: Sole

Mobile, Online, or Brick & Mortar: Online

Potential products to upsell: Books, courses.

Chapter 11
What Next?

Now that you've decided what path you want to pursue, you're probably asking yourself—"What next?" Well my friends, what comes next are commitment. You are going to have to devote some time each day to work towards your goal. You must start somewhere, and you have to be educated before you go into any venture. I commend you for picking up this book to read as your first step. Now you need to get specialized information on your chosen entrepreneurial venture.

The Internet offers a vast amount of information on any topic you could ever imagine. Find the best-recommended books on your topic and read those. I suggest not buying the Kindle format, simply so you can highlight on an actual copy and have quick reference when you really need it. Look for courses and certifications on your topic.

If there is already someone doing something similar to what you want to do, reach out to them and pick their brains about their business. Most people don't mind talking about their business to others unless you are direct competition setting up shop across the street from them. Ask them things like start-up costs, how they market, how long did it take the to break even or make a profit, whatever you have questions-about-ask! I'd say topics that may be off-limits would be discussing actual profit numbers – unless of course they voluntarily offer that information.

Networking is also a big factor that helps you with gaining knowledge on a particular subject. Join interest groups that relate to the type of business you want to be in. Check out meet-up.com and specialized groups on Facebook, Twitter, and Linked-In. Just type in the words "nurse entrepreneur" on any of those sites, and you will find other like-minded individuals you can network with.

Other sources for business information can be found here:

Internet

Library

Books

Courses

Local SCORE or SBA chapter

Blogs

Personal Mentor

Podcasts

Webinars

Local Meet-ups

Networking

Volunteering

Pick-up a part-time job in your chosen career to learn more about the business

Glossary of important business terms.

How to ensure your business is profitable

Remember the rule is, no matter what you choose to do for a business, make sure your products and services you offer are going to be profitable! Don't be afraid to charge what you are worth. This is important for you to be able to cover your monthly operating costs and your own salary, especially if you want to retire from nursing and run your business full-time.

Cash is king in business. If you can provide services that are paid for in advance instead of paid upon receipt, you will do much better in the long term. This means if clients pay for their services BEFORE you render them, you have a greater chance of collecting payments than the other way around and having a client skip out in payments after you have done all the work. Work smarter, not harder. You don't want to be in a situation where you have to pursue payment in the court of law. That is too much of a hassle and not good for your monthly cash flow- A.K.A. profits.

One of the most important things you can do before starting your business besides writing a business plan (covered in *You're a Nurse and*

Want to Start a Business? The Complete Guide) is completing a cash flow analysis in an Excel document. Here is a link to a video explaining how to create an Excel cash flow analysis: https://www.youtube.com/watch?v=C5PcUSmfOZU. A cash flow analysis will give you an idea of whether or not your business venture will be profitable before you dive in headfirst, and let you know how much start-up capital you need.

A cash flow analysis details all starting costs and monthly expenses and profits over a certain period of time (3 years is a good number to start). Once your cash flow analysis is complete, you can use this information to include in your business plan.

The number one reason new businesses fail is because business owners underestimate their first year operating expenses. When you start a business, you have to take into account salaries for yourself and employees, payroll taxes, equipment, rent for office or retail locations, etc. Start-up costs are almost always underestimated by new business owners. This is why it is always important to do a cash flow analysis before you start so your business doesn't fall into the statistic of 50 percent of businesses who fail in the first year.

Your cash flow analysis may grow the longer you work on it, meaning you will find hidden expenses you probably never thought of like purchasing toilet paper and paper towels for your bathroom each month if you have an actual office. Each cash flow analysis is going to be different for each business.

Dealing with discouragement

There is going to come a time during your journey to start a business that you become discouraged with the process. It may deal with lack of money, something or someone not moving fast enough, or encountering setbacks you didn't expect. Anything and everything wrong will happen when you first start out. It's just the nature of going into business for yourself. This is why it is imperative for you to do your due diligence before you jump headfirst into business. You want to work out every possible scenario in your head of what could go wrong and how you would handle it. It is impossible to know everything before it happens, but if you plan for what you can foresee, you can save yourself a lot of heartbreak and money in the future.

One aspect of business you may not realize is that you will work very hard at the beginning (you may not be able to get out of working 12-hour shifts just yet!) only it will not be in the hospital working for someone else! It will be working for you. In the beginning, you will hold the title of owner, accountant, human resources, housekeeping, secretary – you get the picture. Until you and your business become established, you will wear many hats.

Working so much can take a toll on your personal relationships with friends and family. You will have to sit down with those important to you and explain you are working very hard to better yourself (and them if you have a family to support), and they will need to be patient. If you have a business that can enlist your spouse or significant other, then they may able to help you out in your venture. You may have to tell your buddies you can't hang out every weekend, but remember to take time out for yourself during this time so you don't become burned out.

If you feel your motivation for your business waning, take a step back and ask yourself exactly why you want to go into business for yourself and what your motivation is. These are two important questions to ask. If your reasons are not the right ones, it will be easy for you to get frustrated and give up. At this point, you need to really decide if owning a business is right for you. Success does not come easy, and you're going to have to work hard for it if you're looking for the easy way out, then business ownership is not for you.

Another way to avoid disappointment in business is to time your entry in the market to the best of your ability. This means not jumping into something without doing your homework on the market, without having enough working capital, or without having a plan. This also means being aware of when to go into business for as well. Sometimes opportunities present themselves, and we don't take them for some reason or another. Be aware and be open, you never know when an opportunity may present itself.

How to Raise Capital for Your Business

Coming up with enough money for business ventures causes much angst and anxiety for people, with them eventually abandoning their business idea altogether simply because of the money. I know it may sound insurmountable, but do not let the money issue stop you. Where there's a will, there's a way.

I know the idea of getting another idea or working overtime sounds trite, but this is the first option I would pursue. It's the easiest option and offers the least risk. Aside from picking up extra hours, you could ask to borrow money from friends and family, start small with your business with what you have now and expand later, borrow from your retirement accounts, or borrow from the bank. If you have a novel idea, use a platform like Kickstarter or GoFundMe. If necessary, rent out a room in your home. You can do many things to build money for your business. There are pros and cons of all of these options and a certain risk level as well.

Whatever way you raise capital for your business, you also need to make sure you have enough personal savings to cover your own living expenses for at minimum 6 months. When you start out your business will not be profitable for a while, and you want to make sure you can pay your bills during that time. The last thing you want to stress about is money in your personal account when you are starting out. When you start out, another thing that may help with the money crunch is keeping your day job for until you can afford to quit and go full time in your own business. Your days are going to be long in the beginning, but your hard work will pay off in the long term.

If you apply for a business loan, the bank is going to want to see an "additional" source of income, meaning your job or a substantial savings account. Your spouse's income would meet this requirement for you as well. But if you're a single gal (or guy) like me then you're going to have to save as much as possible since you don't have a second person with an income in the family. The bank wants this simply because they know most new businesses are not profitable, and they don't want to see you fail because that means they lose money!

I hope this book has enlightened you on some business ideas for nurses. Of course, this list is not all-inclusive of everything a nurse can do in business, but hopefully it gets the wheels churning on your journey. Don't have fear when starting your own business because many others before you have done it and many others who haven't will admire your guts for doing so.

About the Author

Nachole Johnson is a nurse practitioner who loves educating and inspiring other nurses to succeed in life. She has authored numerous blogs and articles for nursing sites and is the author of *You're a Nurse and Want to Start Your Own Business? The Complete Guide.* She is also CEO of Renursing Career Consulting, a company dedicated to empowering nurses. Learn more at (Link to Amazon Author Page)

Other Books By Nachole Johnson

You're a Nurse and Want to Start Your Own Business? The Complete Guide. Available at https://www.amazon.com/dp/B00H4OVHKC/

Made in United States
Troutdale, OR
02/25/2025